CHAIR YOGA FOR SENIORS

10 Minutes A Day Workout for Flexibility, Balance, and Mobility Improvement

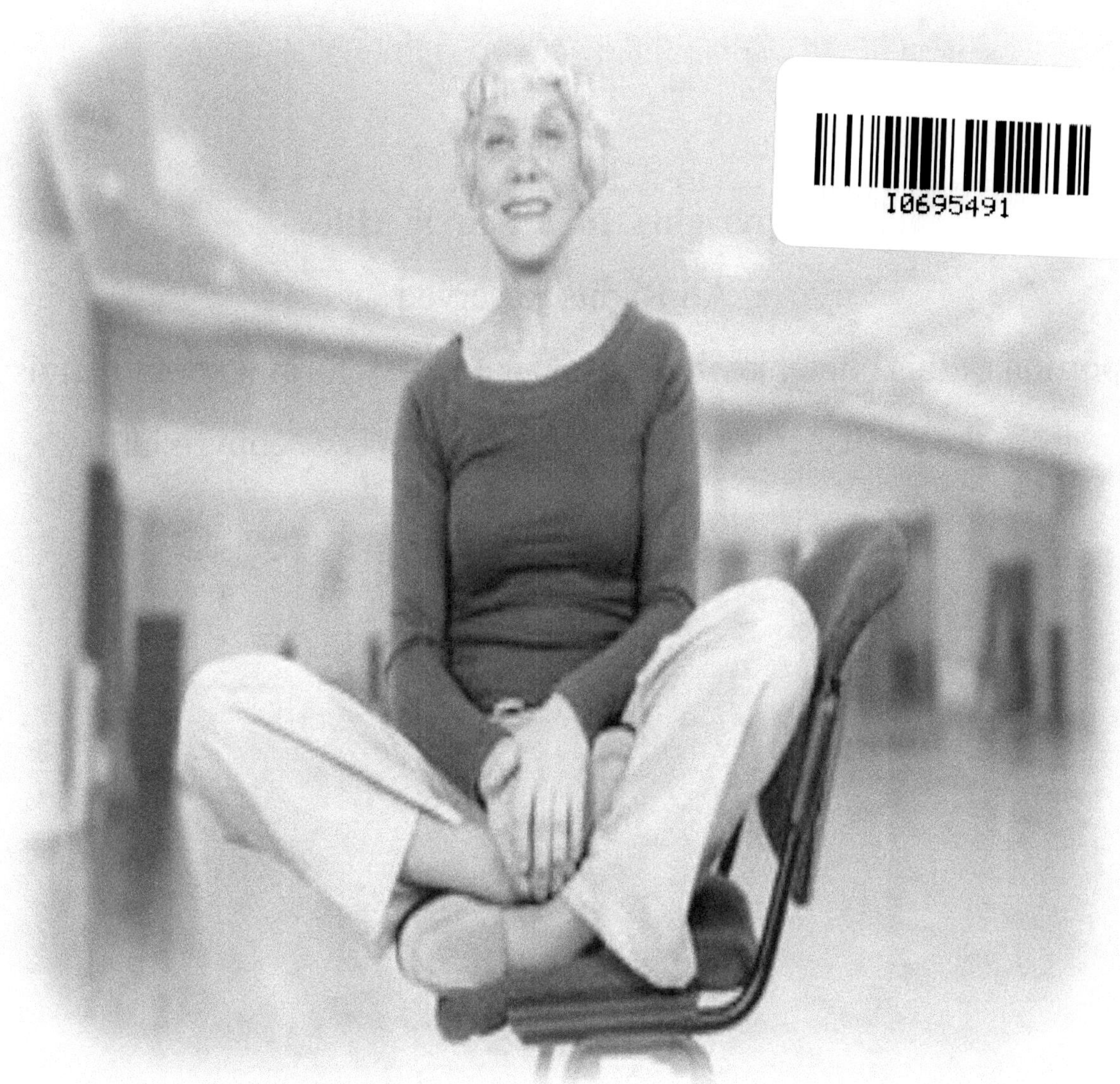

Dr. Laurie Miles

TABLE OF CONTENTS

EXCLUSIVE BONUS OFFER FOR PAPERBACK PURCHASE

As a special bonus for purchasing "Chair Yoga for Seniors - 10 Minutes A Day Workout for Flexibility, Balance, and Mobility Improvement", readers will gain access to an exclusive series of life-changing instructional videos. These meticulously crafted videos are led by a team of seasoned fitness instructors and yoga experts, renowned for their expertise in senior wellness and holistic fitness.

Through this comprehensive video series, you will be able to:

- Immerse yourself in dynamic and engaging chair yoga routines, led by experienced instructors with a deep understanding of seniors' unique needs and abilities.
- Follow along with clear and well-illustrated demonstrations of each exercise, ensuring a seamless and enjoyable learning experience from the comfort of your own home.
- Elevate your practice with personalized tips and guidance, fostering a deeper connection to your body, breath, and inner well-being.
- Embrace a transformative journey towards enhanced flexibility, improved balance, and increased mobility, guided by a team of experts dedicated to your holistic well-being and vitality.

Don't pass up this fantastic opportunity to improve your health and enjoy a life of vitality, balance, and mindful aging.

Get your copy of "Chair Yoga for Seniors - 10 Minutes A Day Workout for Flexibility, Balance, and Mobility Improvement" today and discover chair yoga's revolutionary potential. Remember, the special bonus video series should not be overlooked.

Improve your practice, strengthen your connection to comprehensive well-being, and begin on a transforming path toward a life of resilience and joy. Get your book now and start your journey to fitness and energy.

P.S: Find the QR code and access link to the bonus at the last page of this book.

Introduction

Welcome, dear seniors, to the invigorating and accessible realm of chair yoga! In this transformative journey, we delve into the art of gentle exercises and mindful movements designed to enhance your well-being. Regardless of your mobility or fitness level, chair yoga opens a doorway to a world where you can foster your flexibility, improve your balance, and revitalize your mobility with ease. Embrace this opportunity to embark on a rejuvenating path that celebrates the vitality of your golden years.

The Importance of Flexibility, Balance, and Mobility in Aging Gracefully

As we gracefully age, maintaining our physical flexibility, balance, and mobility becomes increasingly vital. These pillars form the bedrock of our independence and overall quality of life. Preserving flexibility allows us to move with fluidity and ease, ensuring that our daily tasks remain manageable and enjoyable. Sustaining a strong sense of balance provides the foundation for stability and confidence, guarding against potential falls and injuries. Similarly, nurturing mobility empowers us to engage actively with the world around us, fostering a sense of freedom and empowerment that transcends age.

Investigating the Advantages of Chair Yoga for Senior Health and Well-Being

Chair yoga appears as a ray of hope, providing a slew of advantages tailored exclusively to the needs of elders. Chair yoga, with its gentle yet effective exercises, serves as a conduit for increasing flexibility, improving balance, and increasing mobility. Aside from the physical benefits, this practice promotes cerebral clarity, emotional balance, and a profound sense of inner calm. Seniors who practice chair yoga might enjoy better posture, increased energy, and a revitalized enthusiasm for life. Let us investigate the extraordinary ways in which chair yoga can provide joy, vigor, and comprehensive well-being to our older years.

Let us celebrate the art of aging gracefully and living life to the fullest by unlocking the astonishing potential of chair yoga with an open heart and a readiness to embark on this transforming path.

CHAPTER 1

Understanding Senior Health

As we begin our adventure into the world of chair yoga, it is critical that we first have a thorough awareness of senior health. In this chapter, we will delve into the complexities of senior physical well-being, deconstructing the prevalent flexibility issues that seniors have, the difficulty related with balance, and the mobility limitations that might occur during the golden years.

Common Flexibility Issues in Seniors

Being flexible means that our muscles and joints can move in all the ways they are supposed to. It is a fundamental aspect of physical health that often declines with age. Let's delve into the common flexibility issues that seniors encounter and how chair yoga can be the key to addressing these concerns.

Stiffness and Joint Discomfort: As we age, it is not uncommon to experience stiffness in our muscles and joints. This stiffness can be attributed to a variety of factors, including a reduction in the synovial fluid that lubricates the joints and the natural wear and tear of cartilage. Such stiffness can hinder daily activities and lead to discomfort.

Muscle Tightness: The tightening of muscles is a prevalent issue in seniors. It can result from a sedentary lifestyle, inadequate hydration, or even an accumulation of scar tissue from previous injuries. This tightness can limit your range of motion, making it challenging to perform even simple tasks.

Reduced Range of Motion: Seniors often find that their range of motion gradually diminishes over time. This decline can affect their ability to reach, bend, and twist, impacting their day-to-day activities and overall quality of life.

Arthritis: Arthritis is a common condition among seniors, affecting the joints and causing pain and inflammation. It can significantly restrict flexibility and mobility, making it more challenging to engage in physical activities.

Challenges with Balance for Seniors

Balance is a vital component of senior health, as it influences the ability to stand, walk, and move with stability and confidence. The aging process can introduce various challenges related to balance. Let's examine these issues and understand how chair yoga can help improve balance.

Loss of Muscle Mass: A decline in muscle mass, known as sarcopenia, is a natural consequence of aging. This loss of muscle strength can affect balance, making seniors more prone to falls.

Inner Ear Changes: The inner ear plays a significant role in our balance system. As we age, changes in the inner ear's structure and function can result in dizziness and a sense of unsteadiness.

Vision Impairment: Age-related vision problems can affect depth perception and spatial awareness, making it more challenging to maintain balance and navigate through the environment.

Medication Side Effects: Many seniors take medications that can have side effects, including dizziness and lightheadedness, which can further compromise balance.

Mobility Concerns in Senior Living

Mobility encompasses the ability to move freely and independently. It is crucial for maintaining an active and fulfilling lifestyle. However, seniors may face various mobility concerns that can impact their daily lives. Let's delve into these concerns and understand how chair yoga can be a powerful tool for enhancing mobility.

Joint Issues: Joint problems, such as osteoarthritis, can lead to pain and stiffness, affecting the ability to move comfortably. These issues can limit mobility and make activities like walking and climbing stairs challenging.

Chronic Conditions: Seniors may grapple with chronic conditions like diabetes or heart disease, which can influence mobility by causing fatigue and discomfort.

Inactivity: A sedentary lifestyle can contribute to muscle weakness and reduced mobility. Many seniors lead relatively inactive lives, which can lead to a decline in overall physical functionality.

Fear of Falling: A significant concern for many seniors is the fear of falling, which can lead to a lack of confidence in moving around. This fear can become a barrier to maintaining an active lifestyle.

In the next chapters, we will look at how chair yoga can be used to address these typical difficulties. Chair yoga, with its gentle movements and holistic approach to senior health, provides a road to improved flexibility, improved balance, and increased mobility, ensuring that our golden years are full of vitality and well-being.

CHAPTER 2

The Advantages of Chair Yoga

As we dig deeper into the world of chair yoga, it is critical to recognize the enormous benefits that this practice may provide for seniors. In this chapter, we will look at how chair yoga can help you improve your flexibility, balance, and mobility while also cultivating a holistic sense of well-being and vitality.

How Chair Yoga Helps Flexibility

Chair yoga serves as a gentle yet potent tool for enhancing flexibility, ensuring that seniors can move with greater ease and comfort in their daily lives. Let's delve into the ways in which chair yoga fosters and nurtures flexibility, enabling seniors to maintain a sense of fluidity and freedom in their movements.

Gentle Stretching: Chair yoga incorporates a series of gentle stretching exercises that help to loosen the muscles and improve their elasticity. These stretches are specifically designed to be accessible and safe for seniors, allowing them to gradually enhance their flexibility without experiencing discomfort or strain.

Joint Mobility: By encouraging a full range of motion for the joints, chair yoga helps to combat stiffness and maintain joint health. The gentle movements involved in chair yoga target various joints, including those in the shoulders, hips, and spine, fostering flexibility and preventing the onset of stiffness or restricted movement.

Improved Circulation: The controlled breathing techniques and mindful movements practiced in chair yoga promote healthy blood flow throughout the body. This enhanced circulation contributes to better muscle function and flexibility, facilitating the delivery of essential nutrients and oxygen to the muscles and joints.

Pain Management: For seniors grappling with chronic pain or discomfort, chair yoga can serve as a means of managing and alleviating their symptoms. The gentle stretching and movement exercises can help to reduce muscle tension and alleviate joint pain, enabling seniors to enjoy a greater sense of comfort and flexibility in their bodies.

<u>Improving Balance through Chair Yoga</u>

Balance is a cornerstone of physical well-being, influencing our ability to move with stability and confidence. Chair yoga serves as a remarkable tool for improving balance, helping seniors to navigate their surroundings with greater poise and assurance. Let's explore how chair yoga cultivates and refines balance, empowering seniors to move with grace and security.

Core Strengthening: Chair yoga incorporates exercises that target the core muscles, which play a pivotal role in maintaining balance and stability. By strengthening the core, chair yoga helps to improve posture and support the body's equilibrium, enabling seniors to stand and move with greater steadiness and control.

Enhanced Proprioception: Proprioception, the body's ability to sense its position in space, is crucial for maintaining balance. Chair yoga encourages mindful movements and sensory awareness, helping seniors to refine their proprioceptive abilities and develop a heightened sense of balance and coordination.

Focused Breathing Techniques: The incorporation of specific breathing techniques in chair yoga fosters a sense of mindfulness and focus, which are integral to maintaining balance. By cultivating a deep connection between breath and movement, chair yoga enables seniors to enhance their concentration and equilibrium, promoting a greater sense of stability and control.

Postural Alignment: Chair yoga emphasizes the importance of proper postural alignment, guiding seniors to maintain a balanced and aligned stance throughout the practice. This focus on alignment extends beyond the yoga session, encouraging seniors to adopt better posture in their daily activities, thereby reducing the risk of falls and injuries.

Enhancing Mobility with Chair Yoga

Mobility is a key determinant of independence and vitality in senior living. Chair yoga serves as a transformative tool for enhancing mobility, empowering seniors to move with greater freedom and confidence. Let's delve into how chair yoga promotes and fosters mobility, ensuring that seniors can engage actively with the world around them.

Joint Flexibility: By encouraging gentle movements that target the major joints in the body, chair yoga helps to improve joint flexibility and range of motion. This enhanced joint mobility allows seniors to perform daily activities with greater ease and comfort, fostering a sense of independence and empowerment.

Functional Movement Patterns: Chair yoga incorporates exercises that mimic everyday movements, such as reaching, bending, and twisting, ensuring that seniors can maintain their functional movement patterns. By practicing these movements in a controlled and supportive environment, seniors can refine their mobility and carry out daily tasks with confidence and efficiency.

Muscle Strength and Endurance: The gentle strength-building exercises in chair yoga contribute to the development of muscle strength and endurance, enabling seniors to support their body weight and engage in various physical activities with vigor and resilience. This heightened muscular strength and endurance enhance overall mobility and promote a sense of vitality and well-being.

Pain Reduction and Management: For seniors dealing with chronic pain or discomfort, chair yoga can serve as a valuable tool for pain reduction and management. The controlled and gentle movements involved in chair yoga help to alleviate muscle tension and joint pain, enabling seniors to move more freely and comfortably, thereby enhancing their overall mobility and quality of life.

We will go more into the specific chair yoga movements and routines that address flexibility, balance, and mobility, encouraging seniors to enjoy a life of vitality, well-being, and holistic health in the next chapters.

CHAPTER 3

Starting with Chair Yoga

As we begin our chair yoga journey, it is critical to establish a solid foundation that promotes a safe and productive practice. In this chapter, we'll go over the fundamental actions' seniors should take to get started with chair yoga. We will look at how to prepare the body for chair yoga, offer safety advice and guidelines for a safe practice, and emphasize the need of setting realistic objectives to guarantee a fulfilling and long-term chair yoga experience.

Preparing the Body for Chair Yoga

Preparing the body is a crucial step in ensuring a successful and beneficial chair yoga practice. By taking the time to prepare both physically and mentally, seniors can optimize their readiness for the practice, allowing them to engage with the exercises more effectively and comfortably. Let's delve into the various ways in which seniors can prepare their bodies for chair yoga.

Warm-Up Exercises: Incorporating gentle warm-up exercises before beginning chair yoga helps to prepare the muscles and joints for movement. These warm-up exercises can include simple stretches, shoulder rolls, and wrist rotations, aimed at increasing blood flow and enhancing flexibility.

Mindful Breathing: Practicing mindful breathing exercises can help seniors to center themselves and create a sense of calm and focus before starting the chair yoga practice. Taking a few moments to engage in deep breathing can promote relaxation, reduce stress, and establish a mindful connection between the body and the breath.

Body Awareness: Cultivating an awareness of the body's sensations and limitations is crucial in preparing for chair yoga. Seniors are encouraged to listen to their bodies and identify any areas of tension or discomfort, allowing them to approach the practice with mindfulness and self-care.

Setting Intentions: Setting positive intentions for the chair yoga practice can help seniors to approach the session with a sense of purpose and determination. By focusing on specific goals or aspirations, seniors can infuse their practice with meaning and motivation, fostering a deeper connection to the practice and its potential benefits.

Safety Tips and Guidelines for Seniors

Ensuring the safety and well-being of seniors is of paramount importance when practicing chair yoga. By adhering to essential safety tips and guidelines, seniors can create a secure and supportive environment that facilitates a risk-free and enjoyable practice. Let's explore the key safety tips and guidelines that seniors should consider when engaging in chair yoga.

Consulting a Healthcare Professional: Before starting any new exercise regimen, it is advisable for seniors to consult their healthcare provider or a qualified medical professional. This step is essential in identifying any potential health concerns or limitations that may impact the practice of chair yoga.

Choosing a Suitable Chair: Selecting a stable and sturdy chair that provides adequate support is crucial in ensuring a safe and comfortable chair yoga practice. Seniors should opt for a chair with a straight back and a firm seat, avoiding chairs with wheels or unstable structures that may compromise their safety during the practice.

Avoiding Overexertion: Seniors are encouraged to practice chair yoga at their own pace, avoiding overexertion or pushing themselves beyond their comfort limits. It is essential to listen to the body's signals and respect its boundaries, allowing for gradual progress and an enjoyable practice experience.

Modifying Poses as Needed: Modifying poses to accommodate individual abilities and limitations is a key aspect of practicing chair yoga safely. Seniors should feel empowered to make necessary adjustments to the poses, using props or modifications to ensure their comfort and safety throughout the practice.

Setting Realistic Goals for Chair Yoga Practice

Setting realistic and achievable goals is instrumental in fostering a fulfilling and sustainable chair yoga practice. By establishing clear intentions and aspirations, seniors can stay motivated and focused, ensuring that their chair yoga journey is both rewarding and empowering. Let's explore the significance of setting realistic goals for chair yoga practice and how seniors can approach this process with confidence and enthusiasm.

Identifying Personal Objectives: Seniors are encouraged to reflect on their personal objectives and reasons for engaging in chair yoga. Whether the goal is to improve flexibility, enhance balance, or foster a sense of well-being, clarifying these objectives can provide a sense of direction and purpose throughout the practice.

Embracing Gradual Progress: Embracing the concept of gradual progress is essential in setting realistic goals for chair yoga practice. Seniors should approach the practice with patience and an understanding that positive change takes time. By celebrating small milestones and acknowledging incremental improvements, seniors can maintain a sense of motivation and accomplishment.

Adapting to Individual Needs: Recognizing and adapting to individual needs and limitations is crucial in setting realistic goals for chair yoga practice. Seniors should tailor their practice to accommodate their unique abilities and physical condition, ensuring that their goals are both attainable and tailored to their specific requirements.

Celebrating Achievements: Celebrating achievements, no matter how small, is an integral part of the goal-setting process in chair yoga practice. Seniors are encouraged to acknowledge and celebrate their progress, whether it's an improvement in flexibility, an increase in balance, or a heightened sense of well-being. By acknowledging these achievements, seniors can stay motivated and inspired to continue their chair yoga journey with enthusiasm and determination.

In the following chapters, we will look at the fundamentals of chair yoga, bringing seniors through the stages that will allow them to begin a fulfilling and enriching practice. Seniors can build a strong and sustainable basis for their chair yoga journey by incorporating planning, safety, and realistic goal-setting. This will develop a sense of empowerment, well-being, and holistic health.

CHAPTER 4

Simple Chair Yoga Poses for Flexibility

In this chapter, we'll look at a few easy yet powerful chair yoga postures that target different parts of the body, increasing flexibility and overall well-being. These mild poses are specifically created for seniors to be accessible and safe, allowing them to improve range of motion, relieve stiffness, and promote a sense of energy and comfort. Let us look at three major areas of focus: neck and shoulder stretches, modest back and spine exercises, and arm and leg stretching from a chair.

Neck and Shoulder Stretches

Neck and shoulder stretches play a pivotal role in promoting flexibility and relieving tension in these commonly constricted areas. By incorporating gentle and mindful stretches that target the neck and shoulders, seniors can alleviate stiffness, reduce discomfort, and foster a greater sense of relaxation and ease. Let us explore some simple chair yoga poses that facilitate neck and shoulder stretches.

Neck Tilts:

- ➢ Sit comfortably on the chair with the spine straight and the shoulders relaxed.
- ➢ Slowly tilt the head to the right, aiming to bring the right ear closer to the right shoulder without forcing the movement.

➢ Hold this position for a few deep breaths, feeling a gentle stretch along the left side of the neck.

➢ Repeat on the opposite side to ensure a balanced stretch.

Shoulder Rolls:

➢ Sit with the spine tall and the feet grounded.

➢ Inhale deeply as you roll the shoulders up toward the ears, then exhale as you roll them back and down.

➢ Repeat this movement in a smooth, circular motion, allowing the shoulders to relax and release any built-up tension.

➢ Focus on maintaining a slow and controlled pace, emphasizing the full range of motion for the shoulders.

Upper Trapezius Stretch:

➢ Begin by sitting upright in the chair, ensuring proper posture and alignment.

➢ Place the right hand under the right thigh to stabilize the body.

➢ With the left hand, gently tilt the head towards the right, aiming to bring the left ear closer to the left shoulder.

➢ Feel the stretch along the left side of the neck and upper trapezius muscle.

➢ Hold the stretch for several breaths before switching to the opposite side.

Gentle Back and Spine Movements

Gentle back and spine movements are instrumental in fostering spinal flexibility and promoting a healthy range of motion. By engaging in chair yoga poses that encourage gentle twists, bends, and extensions, seniors can alleviate back stiffness, improve posture, and nurture a sense of spinal comfort and well-being. Let us explore some simple chair yoga poses that facilitate gentle back and spine movements.

Seated Cat-Cow Stretch:
- Sit comfortably on the chair with the feet flat on the ground.
- Put your hands on your thighs to help yourself stay balanced.
- As you inhale, arch the back and lift the chest, allowing the shoulders to roll back gently. This is the cow position.
- As you exhale, round the spine and tuck the chin toward the chest, allowing the shoulders to roll forward. This is the cat position.
- Repeat this gentle, flowing movement for several rounds, synchronizing the breath with the motion of the spine.

Seated Spinal Twist:
- Sit with the spine tall and the feet firmly planted on the ground.
- Place the right hand on the outside of the left thigh, and the left hand on the back of the chair for support.
- Inhale deeply, elongating the spine, and as you exhale, gently twist the torso to the left, allowing the head to follow the movement.

- ➤ Feel the stretch along the spine and the gentle release of tension.
- ➤ Hold the twist for a few breaths before repeating on the opposite side.

Seated Forward Bend:

- ➤ Begin by sitting at the edge of the chair with the feet hip-width apart.
- ➤ Inhale deeply, lengthening the spine, and as you exhale, hinge at the hips, allowing the torso to fold forward over the legs.
- ➤ Let the arms hang loosely towards the floor, allowing the head and neck to relax.
- ➤ Feel the gentle stretch along the spine and the back of the legs.
- ➤ Hold this position for several breaths, focusing on maintaining a sense of relaxation and ease.

Stretching the Arms and Legs from a Chair

Stretching the arms and legs from a chair serves as a dynamic and accessible way to promote flexibility and improve circulation in the limbs. By incorporating simple chair yoga poses that target the arms and legs, seniors can enhance their range of motion, alleviate muscle tension, and foster a sense of vitality and well-being. Let us explore some straightforward chair yoga poses that facilitate stretching the arms and legs.

Seated Leg Extensions:

> ➢ Sit with the spine tall and the feet flat on the floor.

> ➢ Extend the right leg forward, pointing the toes towards the ceiling.

> ➢ Flex the foot, engaging the muscles in the leg.

> ➢ Hold the position for a few breaths, feeling the stretch along the back of the leg. Lower the leg back to the ground and repeat with the left leg.

> ➢ Focus on maintaining a smooth and controlled movement, emphasizing the extension and flexion of the legs.

Seated Eagle Arms:

> ➢ Sit comfortably on the chair with the spine tall and the feet grounded.

> ➢ Extend the arms forward at shoulder height, then cross the right arm over the left, bringing the palms to touch. If possible, intertwine the forearms and press the palms together.

> ➢ Lift the elbows slightly, feeling the stretch between the shoulder blades.

> ➢ Hold this position for several breaths before releasing and repeating the cross with the left arm over the right.

Ankle Circles:

> ➢ Sit with the spine tall and the feet flat on the ground.

> ➢ Lift the right foot slightly off the floor and begin to rotate the ankle in a circular motion, first clockwise and then counterclockwise.

➢ Focus on making the circles as fluid and controlled as possible, allowing the movement to be gentle and effortless.

➢ Lower the right foot back to the ground and repeat the ankle circles with the left foot.

➢ Pay attention to any areas of tightness or discomfort, adjusting the movement as needed.

Seniors can encourage increased flexibility, relieve stiffness, and generate a profound sense of well-being and comfort by including these basic chair yoga postures into their daily practice. These gentle and approachable poses can help seniors enjoy their golden years with a sense of empowerment and overall wellness by cultivating physical health and vitality.

CHAPTER 5

Chair Yoga for Improving Balance

In this chapter, we will look at the life-changing impact of chair yoga in improving balance in seniors. We will go over a series of balancing exercises that develop stability and coordination, as well as chair yoga to strengthen the core and emphasize the need of improving stability and coordination to nurture a greater sense of equilibrium and confidence. These simple and effective chair yoga practices can help seniors maintain physical well-being and manage their everyday lives with grace and assurance.

Balancing Exercises for Seniors (3 Poses)

Balancing exercises play a pivotal role in improving stability and preventing falls, particularly among seniors. By incorporating specific chair yoga poses that target balance, seniors can cultivate a greater sense of equilibrium and poise, enabling them to move with confidence and security. Let us explore some simple chair yoga poses that facilitate balancing exercises for seniors.

Single Leg Stance:

> ➢ Sit comfortably on the chair with the spine tall and the feet flat on the floor.
> ➢ Lift the right foot slightly off the ground and balance on the left foot, keeping the right knee bent.
> ➢ Hold this position for a few breaths, focusing on maintaining stability and a steady breath.
> ➢ Switch to balancing on the right foot to ensure equal engagement on both sides. If you need to, lean on the back of the chair for support.

Warrior III Variation:

> ➢ Begin by sitting at the edge of the chair with the feet hip-width apart.
> ➢ Extend the arms forward at shoulder height and hinge at the hips, allowing the torso to lean forward.
> ➢ Lift the right leg back, parallel to the floor, while maintaining a straight line from the head to the extended right foot.
> ➢ Engage the core and focus on maintaining balance and stability.
> ➢ Hold this position for several breaths before switching to the left leg.

Tree Pose with Chair Support:

> ➢ Stand behind the chair and place one hand on the back of the chair for support.

- Shift the weight onto the left leg and lift the right foot, placing the sole of the right foot on the inner left thigh or calf.
- Find a focal point to help maintain balance, and bring the hands to the heart center or extend them overhead.
- Hold this position for several breaths, feeling the grounding connection with the standing leg and the uplifted energy in the body.

<u>Strengthening the Core through Chair Yoga (3 Poses)</u>

A strong and stable core serves as a foundation for maintaining balance and promoting overall physical well-being. By engaging in chair yoga poses that target core strength, seniors can foster a sense of stability and support, enabling them to navigate their daily activities with confidence and ease. Let us explore some simple chair yoga poses that focus on strengthening the core.

- **Seated Spinal Twist:**
- Sit with the spine tall and the feet firmly planted on the ground.
- Place the right hand on the outside of the left thigh, and the left hand on the back of the chair for support.
- Inhale deeply, elongating the spine, and as you exhale, gently twist the torso to the left, allowing the head to follow the movement.
- Feel the engagement of the core muscles as you deepen the twist.
- Hold the twist for a few breaths before repeating on the opposite side.

Boat Pose Variation:

 ➢ Begin by sitting at the edge of the chair with the feet flat on the ground.
 ➢ Hold onto the sides of the chair for support.
 ➢ Lean back slightly, engaging the core, and lift the legs a few inches off the ground, keeping the knees bent.
 ➢ Find a balance between the sitting bones and the engagement of the abdominal muscles.
 ➢ Hold this position for several breaths, feeling the strengthening and stabilizing effect on the core.

Plank Pose on the Chair:

 ➢ Sit at the edge of the chair with the hands placed on the seat and the fingers pointing towards the knees.
 ➢ Walk the feet back, extending the legs and aligning the body in a straight line from the head to the heels.
 ➢ Engage the abdominal muscles and hold this position for several breaths, focusing on maintaining a strong and stable core.
 ➢ Use the chair for support and stability as needed.

Enhancing stability and coordination is crucial for maintaining a sense of confidence and assurance in daily activities. By integrating chair yoga poses that emphasize stability and coordination, seniors can refine their motor skills, promote spatial awareness, and foster a greater sense of balance and control. Let us explore some simple chair yoga poses that facilitate stability and coordination.

Extended Hand-to-Big-Toe Pose:
- Sit with the spine tall and the feet firmly planted on the ground.
- Extend the right leg forward, keeping the foot flexed, and reach the right hand to hold onto the right big toe.
- Engage the core and find a balance between the sitting bones and the extended leg.
- Hold this position for several breaths, feeling the connection between the extended leg and the stability in the core.
- Repeat on the opposite side.

Cross Crawl Exercise:
- Sit comfortably on the chair with the spine tall and the feet flat on the ground.

- In a slow and controlled motion, lift the right knee towards the chest as you simultaneously bring the left elbow towards the knee.
- Return to the starting position and repeat the movement on the opposite side, bringing the right elbow towards the left knee.
- Continue this cross-crawl motion in a rhythmic and coordinated pattern, emphasizing the engagement of the core and the fluidity of movement.

Chair Warrior II Pose:

- Sit with the spine tall and the feet planted firmly on the ground.
- Extend the right leg out to the side, keeping the foot grounded.
- Rotate the torso to the right, allowing the right arm to reach forward and the left arm to extend behind, creating a line of energy from fingertip to fingertip.
- Engage the core and find stability in the legs as you hold this position for several breaths.
- Repeat on the opposite side.

Seniors can improve their balance, strengthen their core, and perfect their stability and coordination by including chair yoga techniques into their daily routine. These simple and powerful chair yoga poses are great tools for instilling confidence and assurance in seniors, allowing them to go about their everyday lives with grace, poise, and a profound sense of well-being and energy.

CHAPTER 6

Chair Yoga Routine for Mobility Enhancement

Increasing Joint Flexibility and Range of Motion (3 Exercises)

Increasing joint flexibility and range of motion is vital for maintaining an active and fulfilling lifestyle. By incorporating specific chair yoga poses that target joint mobility, seniors can alleviate stiffness, reduce discomfort, and foster a greater sense of freedom and ease in their movements. Let us explore some simple chair yoga exercises that promote joint flexibility and range of motion.

Ankle Rolls and Flexes:

- ➢ Sit comfortably on the chair with the spine tall and the feet flat on the ground.
- ➢ Lift the right foot slightly off the floor and begin to rotate the ankle in a circular motion, first clockwise and then counterclockwise.
- ➢ Focus on making the circles as fluid and controlled as possible, allowing the movement to be gentle and effortless.
- ➢ Repeat the ankle rolls and flexes with the left foot, emphasizing the importance of maintaining mobility and flexibility in the ankles.

Wrist Circles:

> ➤ Sit with the spine tall and the arms resting comfortably on the thighs.
> ➤ Begin to rotate the wrists in a circular motion, first clockwise and then counterclockwise.
> ➤ Focus on creating smooth and controlled circles, allowing the wrists to move freely and comfortably.
> ➤ Pay attention to any areas of tightness or discomfort, adjusting the movement as needed to promote joint flexibility and alleviate stiffness.

Hip Circles:

> ➤ Sit at the edge of the chair with the feet firmly planted on the ground.
> ➤ Place the hands on the hips for support.
> ➤ Begin to rotate the hips in a circular motion, first clockwise and then counterclockwise.
> ➤ Emphasize the fluidity and ease of movement, allowing the hips to release any tension or tightness.
> ➤ Focus on promoting mobility and range of motion in the hips, fostering a greater sense of comfort and ease in daily activities.

<u>**Exercises to Improve Walking and Movement (3 Exercises)**</u>

Improving walking and movement is instrumental in fostering independence and vitality for seniors. By integrating chair yoga exercises that focus on enhancing gait and mobility, seniors can refine their motor skills, promote balance, and foster a greater sense of confidence and assurance in their daily movements. Let us explore some simple chair yoga exercises that facilitate improved walking and movement.

Seated Marching:

➤ Sit comfortably on the chair with the spine tall and the feet flat on the ground. Begin to lift one knee towards the chest, then lower it back to the ground and repeat with the opposite leg.

➤ Focus on creating a rhythmic and controlled movement, allowing the arms to swing naturally with each step.

➤ Emphasize the engagement of the core and the fluidity of the marching motion to promote coordination and enhance walking ability.

Heel-Toe Raises:

➤ Sit with the spine tall and the feet flat on the ground.

➤ Begin to lift the heels off the floor, balancing on the balls of the feet, then lower the heels back down.

➤ Repeat this motion several times, emphasizing the engagement of the calf muscles and the stability in the ankles.

➤ Transition to lifting the toes off the ground while keeping the heels planted, focusing on promoting strength and flexibility in the toes and the front of the feet.

Seated Side Steps:

➤ Sit comfortably on the chair with the spine tall and the feet firmly planted on the ground.

➤ Begin to step the right foot out to the side, then bring it back to the starting position.

➤ Repeat this motion with the left foot, focusing on creating a smooth and controlled side-to-side movement.

➤ Emphasize the engagement of the hip muscles and the stability in the legs to promote balance and coordination in lateral movements.

Enhancing Overall Body Functionality with Chair Yoga (3 Exercises)

Enhancing overall body functionality is essential for fostering a sense of vitality and well-being in seniors. By integrating chair yoga poses that target various areas of the body, seniors can promote muscle strength, improve circulation, and nurture a profound sense of physical and mental wellness. Let us explore some simple chair yoga exercises that enhance overall body functionality.

Seated Sun Salutations:

➢ Sit with the spine tall and the hands resting on the thighs.

➢ Inhale deeply as you raise the arms overhead, then exhale as you lower the arms back down.

➢ Repeat this motion several times, focusing on synchronizing the breath with the movement.

➢ Emphasize the elongation of the spine and the engagement of the shoulder muscles to promote circulation and vitality throughout the body.

Seated Twist and Reach:

➢ Sit with the spine tall and the feet flat on the ground.

➢ Inhale deeply as you lengthen the spine, then exhale as you gently twist the torso to the right, allowing the left hand to reach towards the right knee and the right hand to reach behind the chair.

➢ Hold this position for a few breaths, feeling the gentle twist along the spine. Repeat the twist on the opposite side, emphasizing the engagement of the core and the release of tension in the back muscles.

Seated Mountain Pose:

➢ Sit with the spine tall and the feet grounded.

➢ Inhale deeply as you reach the arms overhead, allowing the palms to touch. Exhale as you lower the arms back down, focusing on maintaining a strong and stable posture.
➢ Repeat this motion several times, emphasizing the extension of the spine and the activation of the core muscles.
➢ Focus on promoting overall body functionality and fostering a sense of balance and vitality.

Seniors can increase their joint flexibility, improve their walking and movement, and boost total body functionality by including these chair yoga activities into their daily practice. These simple and efficient chair yoga exercises are essential tools for promoting physical well-being and empowering elders to live a life of vibrancy, independence, and optimal wellness.

CHAPTER 7

Incorporating Breathing Techniques in Chair Yoga

We will look at the transforming impact of combining breathing methods into chair yoga for seniors in this chapter. We'll go over a series of breathing exercises designed to promote relaxation and stress reduction, establish a link between breath and movement, and improve attention and mental clarity through breath awareness. These simple and powerful breathing practices can help seniors foster emotional well-being and build a profound sense of calm, presence, and inner harmony.

Breathing Exercises for Relaxation and Stress Reduction (3 Exercises)

Breathing exercises serve as a powerful tool for promoting relaxation and reducing stress, allowing seniors to cultivate a sense of calm and tranquility in their daily lives. By integrating specific chair yoga breathing exercises, seniors can alleviate tension, reduce anxiety, and foster a greater sense of emotional well-being. Let us explore some simple breathing techniques that promote relaxation and stress reduction.

Deep Abdominal Breathing:

> Sit comfortably on the chair with the spine tall and the feet flat on the ground. Place just one of your hands on your stomach and the other on your chest. Inhale deeply through the nose, allowing the breath to expand the abdomen and fill the lungs.

> Exhale slowly through the mouth, feeling the gentle contraction of the abdomen.

> Focus on creating a smooth and controlled breath, emphasizing the relaxation of the body and the release of any stress or tension.

Counted Breath Technique:

> Sit with the spine tall and the hands resting comfortably on the thighs.

> Inhale deeply through the nose for a count of four, allowing the breath to fill the lungs completely.

> Hold the breath for a count of four, then exhale slowly through the mouth for a count of six, releasing any tension or discomfort.

> Repeat this cycle several times, focusing on synchronizing the breath with the counts to promote a sense of relaxation and inner peace.

Progressive Muscle Relaxation with Breath:

> Sit comfortably on the chair with the spine tall and the hands resting on the thighs.

- Inhale deeply as you gently tense the muscles in the body, starting from the toes and moving up to the shoulders.
- Hold the tension for a few seconds, then exhale slowly as you release the tension and allow the muscles to relax completely.
- Focus on the connection between the breath and the release of muscle tension, promoting a profound sense of relaxation and stress reduction.

<u>Connecting Breath with Movement for Seniors (3 Exercises)</u>

Connecting breath with movement serves as a fundamental practice in chair yoga, enabling seniors to synchronize their breath with the flow of gentle and mindful movements. By integrating specific chair yoga exercises that emphasize breath awareness, seniors can enhance their physical well-being, promote mindfulness, and foster a deeper connection between the body and the breath. Let us explore some simple chair yoga exercises that facilitate a connection between breath and movement.

Seated Sun Salutations with Breath Awareness:
- Sit with the spine tall and the hands resting on the thighs.
- Inhale deeply as you raise the arms overhead, then exhale as you lower the arms back down.
- Repeat this motion several times, focusing on synchronizing the breath with the movement.

➢ Emphasize the elongation of the spine and the engagement of the shoulder muscles to promote circulation and vitality throughout the body.

Chair Warrior II Pose with Breath Integration:
➢ Sit with the spine tall and the feet firmly planted on the ground.
➢ Extend the right leg out to the side, keeping the foot grounded.
➢ Rotate the torso to the right, allowing the right arm to reach forward and the left arm to extend behind, creating a line of energy from fingertip to fingertip.
➢ Inhale deeply as you lengthen the spine, then exhale as you deepen the pose, focusing on maintaining a strong and steady breath throughout the movement.

Seated Cat-Cow Stretch with Breath Connection:
➢ Sit comfortably on the chair with the feet flat on the ground.
➢ Rest your hands on your thighs for stability.
➢ Inhale deeply as you arch the back and lift the chest, allowing the shoulders to roll back gently. This is the cow position.
➢ Exhale as you round the spine and tuck the chin toward the chest, allowing the shoulders to roll forward. This is the cat position.
➢ Repeat this gentle, flowing movement, focusing on synchronizing the breath with the motion of the spine to promote flexibility and relaxation.

Improving Focus and Mental Clarity through Breath Awareness
(3 Exercises)

Improving focus and mental clarity is essential for nurturing a sense of presence and mindfulness in seniors. By integrating chair yoga practices that emphasize breath awareness, seniors can enhance their cognitive function, promote a sense of mental alertness, and foster a deeper connection to the present moment. Let us explore some simple chair yoga exercises that facilitate breath awareness and improve focus and mental clarity.

Seated Mindful Breathing Meditation:

> Sit comfortably on the chair with the spine tall and the hands resting on the thighs.

> Close the eyes gently and bring the awareness to the natural flow of the breath. Notice the inhalation and exhalation, allowing the breath to guide the attention inward.

> Focus on the sensations of the breath, the rise and fall of the chest, and the gentle rhythm of the inhalation and exhalation.

> Emphasize the cultivation of mindfulness and inner awareness, promoting a sense of mental clarity and peace.

Seated Alternate Nostril Breathing:

> Sit with the spine tall and the hands resting comfortably on the thighs.

- Cover your right nostril with your right thumb and take a deep breath in through your left nostril.
- Cover your left nostril with your ring finger and breathe out through your right nostril.
- Inhale through your right nostril, then close it with your thumb and breathe out through your left nostril.
- Repeat this alternating breath pattern several times, focusing on the balance and harmony between the left and right sides of the body and the mind.

Breath Counting Technique for Concentration:
- Sit with the spine tall and the hands resting on the thighs.
- Inhale deeply through the nose for a count of four, allowing the breath to fill the lungs completely.
- Hold the breath for a count of four, then exhale slowly through the mouth for a count of six, releasing any tension or discomfort.
- Repeat this cycle, focusing on counting the breath to promote concentration and mental clarity.

Seniors can encourage relaxation, cultivate mindfulness, and increase attention and mental clarity by including these breathing methods into their chair yoga practice.

CHAPTER 8

Overcoming Challenges and Staying Motivated

In this chapter, we'll look at the most important tactics for overcoming obstacles and keeping motivated in chair yoga practice for seniors. We'll look at how to deal with setbacks, get support and establish a community, and cultivate a positive mindset for persistent practice. These core characteristics of resilience and motivation are critical tools in cultivating a sense of perseverance, empowerment, and holistic well-being for seniors embarking on their yoga journey.

Dealing with Setbacks in Chair Yoga Practice

Dealing with setbacks is an integral part of the chair yoga journey, as seniors navigate physical limitations, health concerns, and emotional barriers that may impede their practice. By cultivating resilience and a proactive approach to addressing setbacks, seniors can develop the inner strength and fortitude necessary to overcome challenges and continue their yoga practice with confidence and determination. Let us explore some effective strategies for dealing with setbacks in chair yoga practice.

Adaptive Modification Strategies:

Encouraging seniors to adopt adaptive modification strategies that cater to their current physical abilities and address any setbacks they may encounter during their yoga practice. Introduce alternative chair yoga poses, utilize supportive props, and emphasize gentle and mindful movements that alleviate strain and discomfort. Guide seniors in fostering a sense of adaptability and flexibility in their practice, allowing them to navigate setbacks with grace and resilience.

Mindful Rest and Recovery Practices:

Advocating for the integration of mindful rest and recovery practices into seniors' chair yoga routine, allowing them to prioritize self-care and rejuvenation during challenging times. Introducing relaxation techniques, such as guided meditation, deep breathing exercises, and gentle stretching, that promote a sense of calm and inner peace. Emphasizing the importance of honoring the body's needs and limitations, fostering a nurturing and compassionate approach to self-care and well-being.

Goal Realignment and Self-Compassion:

Facilitating open and honest discussions with seniors regarding their goals and expectations for their chair yoga practice, encouraging them to realign their aspirations and priorities in light of any setbacks they may face. Foster a sense of self-compassion and understanding, emphasizing that setbacks are a natural part of the journey towards growth and self-improvement. Guide seniors in redefining success based on personal progress and resilience, fostering a positive and empowering mindset that fuels their motivation and determination.

Finding Support and Building a Community

Finding support and building a community play a crucial role in fostering a sense of belonging and encouragement for seniors on their chair yoga journey. By cultivating a supportive network of peers, mentors, and caregivers, seniors can access valuable resources, guidance, and emotional reinforcement that empower them to overcome challenges and maintain a consistent and fulfilling yoga practice. Let us explore some effective strategies for finding support and building a community in chair yoga practice.

Peer Mentorship and Collaboration:
Encouraging seniors to engage in peer mentorship and collaboration, fostering a sense of camaraderie and mutual empowerment within the chair yoga community. Facilitate group discussions, collaborative practice sessions, and shared experiences that promote an atmosphere of inclusivity and encouragement. Emphasize the value of learning from one another, celebrating each other's achievements, and fostering a collective sense of growth and resilience within the community.

Caregiver and Instructor Partnerships:

Fostering strong partnerships between caregivers and chair yoga instructors, creating a supportive and collaborative environment that prioritizes seniors' well-being and progress. Encourage open communication, regular updates, and collaborative goal-setting that aligns with seniors' unique needs and abilities. Promote a holistic and integrated approach to care and instruction that fosters a seamless and empowering chair yoga experience for seniors, ensuring they feel supported and valued in their practice.

Community Engagement and Outreach Initiatives:

Advocate for active community engagement and outreach initiatives that promote chair yoga practice as a holistic and accessible wellness option for seniors of all backgrounds and abilities. Organize community events, workshops, and informational sessions that raise awareness about the benefits of chair yoga and foster a sense of inclusivity and belonging within the broader community. Emphasize the importance of creating a welcoming and supportive environment that encourages seniors to explore and embrace the transformative power of chair yoga practice.

Cultivating a Positive Mindset for Consistent Practice

Cultivating a positive mindset is essential for maintaining a consistent and fulfilling chair yoga practice for seniors. By nurturing an optimistic and resilient outlook, seniors can overcome self-doubt, build self-confidence, and embrace a sense of purpose and fulfillment in their yoga journey. Let us explore some effective strategies for cultivating a positive mindset for consistent chair yoga practice.

Daily Affirmations and Reflections:

Encouraging seniors to practice daily affirmations and reflections that foster a sense of self-confidence and self-worth. Promote positive self-talk, encouraging seniors to acknowledge their progress, resilience, and inner strength. Guiding them in cultivating a positive and empowering internal dialogue that nurtures a sense of optimism and self-acceptance, fostering a consistent and fulfilling chair yoga practice.

Visualization and Goal Setting:

Advocating for the integration of visualization and goal-setting techniques that empower seniors to envision their desired outcomes and aspirations for their chair yoga practice. Encouraging seniors to set specific, achievable goals that align with their personal growth and well-being, and guide them in visualizing themselves succeeding and thriving in their yoga journey. Emphasizing the transformative power of visualization in fostering a sense of purpose and motivation, fueling seniors' commitment to consistent and dedicated practice.

Mindful Gratitude Practice:

Foster a culture of mindful gratitude within the chair yoga community, encouraging seniors to express gratitude for their physical abilities, their supportive network, and the transformative impact of their yoga practice. Introduce mindful gratitude practices, such as gratitude journaling, acts of kindness, and communal appreciation circles, that promote a sense of interconnectedness and emotional well-being. Emphasize the nurturing and empowering effects of gratitude in cultivating a positive and resilient mindset for consistent chair yoga practice.

Seniors can build a sense of resilience, camaraderie, and optimism in their chair yoga practice by applying these tactics for overcoming hurdles and staying motivated. These fundamental principles of adaptation, support, and a positive outlook are critical tools for fostering physical and emotional well-being and encouraging seniors to live a life of energy, growth, and holistic health.

CHAPTER 9

Chair Yoga as a Lifestyle for Long-Term Well-being

In this final chapter, we will look at the life-changing effect of chair yoga as a lifestyle for seniors' long-term well-being. We will look at how to incorporate chair yoga into daily activities, how to maintain a healthy and active lifestyle, and how to embrace wellness and mindful aging through chair yoga. These core components of chair yoga as a holistic and sustainable lifestyle are important tools in developing physical vitality, emotional resilience, and a profound sense of well-being for seniors on their path to long-term health and joy.

Integrating Chair Yoga into Daily Activities

Integrating chair yoga into daily activities is instrumental in fostering a seamless and accessible yoga practice that complements seniors' lifestyle and routines. By incorporating simple and effective chair yoga poses and breathing techniques into their daily schedule, seniors can promote physical flexibility, emotional balance, and mental clarity, enhancing their overall well-being and vitality. Let us explore some effective strategies for integrating chair yoga into daily activities.

Morning Chair Yoga Rituals:

Encouraging seniors to kickstart their day with a gentle and invigorating chair yoga routine that promotes flexibility and mindfulness. Introduce a series of simple stretches, breathing exercises, and mindful movements that energize the body and awaken the mind, setting a positive and empowering tone for the day ahead. Emphasize the importance of cultivating a morning chair yoga ritual that fosters a sense of presence and vitality, preparing seniors for a day filled with purpose and well-being.

Chair Yoga Breaks Throughout the Day:

Advocating for the implementation of brief chair yoga breaks throughout the day, allowing seniors to alleviate stress, reduce tension, and reinvigorate their mind and body. Introduce a series of quick and accessible chair yoga poses and breathing exercises that can be seamlessly integrated into seniors' daily activities, whether at home, in the workplace, or during leisure time. Emphasize the transformative power of chair yoga breaks in promoting relaxation, rejuvenation, and emotional well-being, fostering a balanced and fulfilling daily routine.

Evening Chair Yoga Rituals for Relaxation:

Encourage seniors to wind down their day with a calming and soothing evening chair yoga ritual that promotes relaxation and peaceful sleep. Introduce gentle stretches, restorative poses, and mindfulness practices that promote physical release and emotional tranquility, allowing seniors to unwind and reflect on the day's experiences. Emphasize the importance of cultivating an evening chair yoga ritual that fosters a sense of inner peace and rejuvenation, preparing seniors for a restful and revitalizing night's sleep.

Staying Healthy and Fit as You Grow Older

Maintaining a healthy and active lifestyle is essential for promoting longevity, vitality, and holistic well-being for seniors. By embracing a balanced and inclusive approach to physical activity, nutrition, and self-care, seniors can cultivate a sense of vitality and resilience that transcends age and fosters a fulfilling and meaningful life. Let us explore some effective strategies for maintaining a healthy and active lifestyle as a senior.

Inclusive Physical Activity Regimens:
Advocate for the implementation of inclusive and accessible physical activity regimens that cater to seniors' unique needs and abilities. Introduce a variety of low-impact exercises, such as chair yoga, gentle walking, and water aerobics, that promote cardiovascular health, muscle strength, and joint flexibility. Emphasize the importance of tailoring physical activity regimens to seniors' comfort and enjoyment, fostering a sustainable and empowering approach to maintaining an active and fulfilling lifestyle.

Balanced and Nutritious Diet Plans: Encourage seniors to adopt balanced and nutritious diet plans that prioritize whole foods, lean proteins, and essential nutrients that support overall well-being and vitality. Introduce a variety of fresh fruits, vegetables, whole grains, and lean proteins that provide essential vitamins and minerals for maintaining healthy body function and promoting a strong immune system. Emphasize the importance of mindful eating and portion control, fostering a nourishing and sustainable approach to maintaining a healthy and active lifestyle.

Holistic Self-Care Practices:

Foster the integration of holistic self-care practices that promote emotional well-being, stress management, and overall mind-body balance for seniors. Introduce relaxation techniques, such as meditation, deep breathing exercises, and aromatherapy, that alleviate tension, reduce anxiety, and foster a sense of inner peace and tranquility. Emphasize the importance of prioritizing self-care as an integral part of maintaining a healthy and active lifestyle, fostering a holistic and empowering approach to well-being and longevity.

Embracing Wellness and Mindful Aging through Chair Yoga

Embracing wellness and mindful aging through the practice of chair yoga is instrumental in fostering a sense of purpose, fulfillment, and holistic well-being for seniors. By cultivating mindfulness, self-compassion, and gratitude, seniors can embrace the transformative power of chair yoga as a lifelong journey towards vitality, resilience, and inner harmony. Let us explore some effective strategies for embracing wellness and mindful aging through chair yoga.

Cultivation of Mindful Awareness:

Encourage seniors to cultivate mindful awareness in their chair yoga practice, fostering a deeper connection to their breath, body, and inner sensations. Guide them in embracing the present moment with an open and compassionate attitude, allowing them to experience each chair yoga pose and breathing technique with a sense of curiosity and non-judgment. Emphasize the transformative power of mindful awareness in fostering emotional resilience, self-acceptance, and a profound sense of inner peace and well-being.

Integration of Self-Compassion and Gratitude:

Foster a culture of self-compassion and gratitude within the chair yoga community, encouraging seniors to nurture a positive and nurturing relationship with themselves and others. Advocate for the integration of self-compassion practices, such as positive affirmations, acts of self-care, and self-appreciation, that promote a sense of inner worth and emotional resilience. Emphasize the transformative power of gratitude in fostering a sense of interconnectedness, joy, and fulfillment in the journey of mindful aging and holistic well-being.

Exploration of Holistic Wellness Modalities:

Encourage seniors to explore various holistic wellness modalities that complement their chair yoga practice, such as aromatherapy, sound therapy, and mindfulness-based stress reduction techniques. Introduce a variety of wellness practices that promote emotional balance, physical vitality, and spiritual alignment, allowing seniors to cultivate a comprehensive and integrated approach to their overall well-being and mindful aging. Emphasize the importance of embracing a holistic and inclusive wellness journey that nurtures the mind, body, and spirit, fostering a profound and sustainable sense of vitality and resilience.

Seniors can cultivate a sense of vitality, purpose, and holistic well-being that transcends age and fosters a fulfilling and meaningful life by implementing these strategies for incorporating chair yoga into daily activities, maintaining a healthy and active lifestyle, and embracing wellness and mindful aging. These core concepts of holistic wellness and mindful aging are critical tools for cultivating physical and emotional resilience and encouraging seniors to enjoy a life of vitality, growth, and long-term well-being.

Conclusion

As we draw to the end of this fascinating tour of the world of chair yoga for seniors, it is clear that this holistic practice has enormous promise for building physical well-being, mental resilience, and a profound sense of holistic vitality. We have discussed the importance of flexibility, balance, and mobility in seniors' overall health and quality of life throughout the chapters, emphasizing the transforming power of chair yoga in addressing these important areas of concern. We have seen the remarkable influence that chair yoga can have on seniors' well-being and their journey towards mindful aging and long-term vitality, from the welcome embrace of chair yoga to the cultivation of a positive mindset and the integration of this practice into daily activities.

Flexibility, an important feature of physical well-being, is a pillar of seniors' mobility and functional independence. We addressed the hurdles they confront by developing a complete understanding of common flexibility concerns in seniors and identified how chair yoga acts as a catalyst for improving joint mobility, muscle flexibility, and general physical resilience. Seniors can uncover a greater sense of freedom, comfort, and fluidity in their movement by engaging in basic chair yoga postures suited to specific areas of difficulty, encouraging them to embrace an active and vibrant existence with confidence and grace.

Balance, a fundamental component of stability and postural control, is critical in the everyday activities and general safety of seniors. We have experienced the transformative impact of creating a strong and solid foundation for physical well-being by digging into the issues connected with balance in seniors and examining the broad spectrum of chair yoga movements designed to promote balance and coordination. Seniors can build a sense of confidence and stability by incorporating chair yoga poses that stress core strength, proprioception, and spatial awareness, allowing them to negotiate their daily routines with grace, resilience, and a heightened sense of awareness.

Mobility, an important aspect in seniors' functional independence and general quality of life, demonstrates their adaptation and perseverance. We have celebrated the profound impact of chair yoga in nurturing a sense of vitality, independence, and holistic health through an exploration of the mobility concerns faced by seniors and the diverse chair yoga routines designed to enhance joint flexibility, promote fluid movement, and foster overall body functionality. Seniors can create a profound sense of well-being and resilience by engaging in specific chair yoga activities that prioritize joint mobility, walking efficiency, and general body functionality, allowing them to enjoy an active and satisfying lifestyle with confidence and enthusiasm.

The benefits of chair yoga are far-reaching and multifaceted, encompassing not only physical well-being but also emotional balance and mental clarity. By unraveling the transformative power of chair yoga in promoting flexibility, improving balance, and enhancing mobility, we have witnessed the profound impact of this practice on seniors' overall health and quality of life. Through the integration of breathing techniques, mindful movement, and self-compassion practices, seniors can foster a deeper connection to their inner resilience, cultivate a profound sense of well-being, and embrace a life of vitality, growth, and mindful aging with grace and dignity.

It is essential to recognize that chair yoga is not merely an exercise routine but a holistic lifestyle that fosters a sense of purpose, resilience, and inner harmony for seniors. By embracing chair yoga as a lifestyle for long-term well-being, seniors can integrate this transformative practice into their daily activities, maintain a healthy and active lifestyle, and cultivate a profound sense of wellness and mindful aging. Through the cultivation of mindfulness, self-compassion, and gratitude, seniors can navigate life's challenges with grace and resilience, fostering a profound sense of purpose and fulfillment that transcends age and empowers them to embrace a life of vitality, growth, and holistic well-being.

As we say goodbye to this educational adventure of chair yoga for elders, let us carry the lessons and insights learned from this journey forward, promoting a culture of inclusivity, empowerment, and holistic well-being for seniors in our communities and beyond. May chair yoga's transformational power continue to serve as a beacon of hope, resilience, and inner harmony for everyone who desire to embrace a life of energy, grace, and mindful aging. With gratitude, compassion, and steadfast support, let us celebrate the remarkable impact of chair yoga on the well-being of seniors and commemorate their journey toward a life of energy, growth, and holistic health.

https://rebrand.ly/chair-yoga-for-seniors

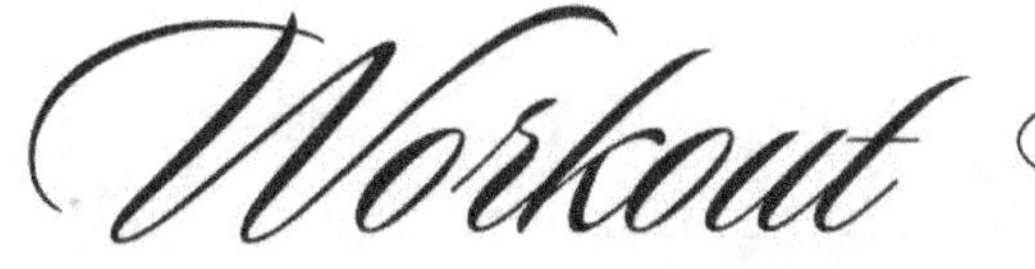 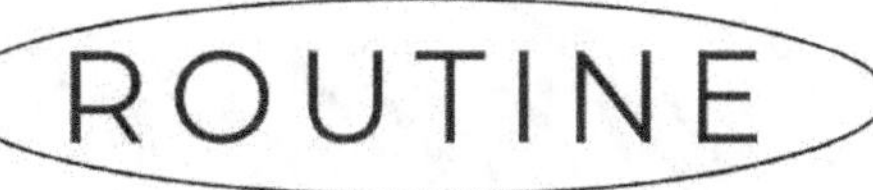

Workout ROUTINE
PLANNER

WEEK ______________

	WORKOUT	SOMETHING TO EAT	MY GOALS
Monday			

	WORKOUT	SOMETHING TO EAT	MY GOALS
Tuesday			

	WORKOUT	SOMETHING TO EAT	MY GOALS
Wednesday			

	WORKOUT	SOMETHING TO EAT	MY GOALS
Thursday			

	WORKOUT	SOMETHING TO EAT	MY GOALS
Friday			

	WORKOUT	SOMETHING TO EAT	MY GOALS
Saturday			

	WORKOUT	SOMETHING TO EAT	MY GOALS
Sunday			

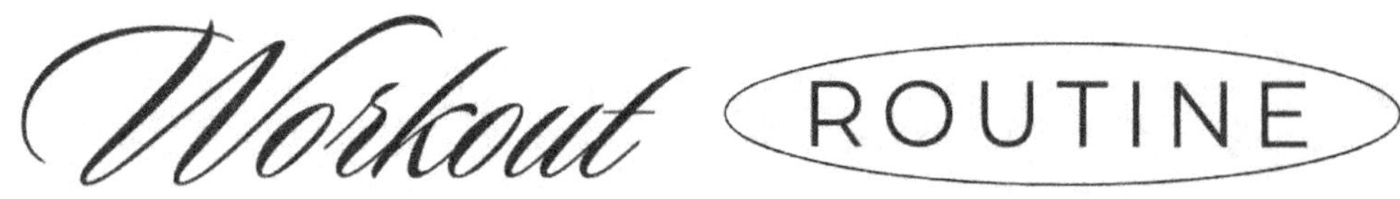

WEEK _______________

	WORKOUT	SOMETHING TO EAT	MY GOALS
Monday			

	WORKOUT	SOMETHING TO EAT	MY GOALS
Tuesday			

	WORKOUT	SOMETHING TO EAT	MY GOALS
Wednesday			

	WORKOUT	SOMETHING TO EAT	MY GOALS
Thursday			

	WORKOUT	SOMETHING TO EAT	MY GOALS
Friday			

	WORKOUT	SOMETHING TO EAT	MY GOALS
Saturday			

	WORKOUT	SOMETHING TO EAT	MY GOALS
Sunday			

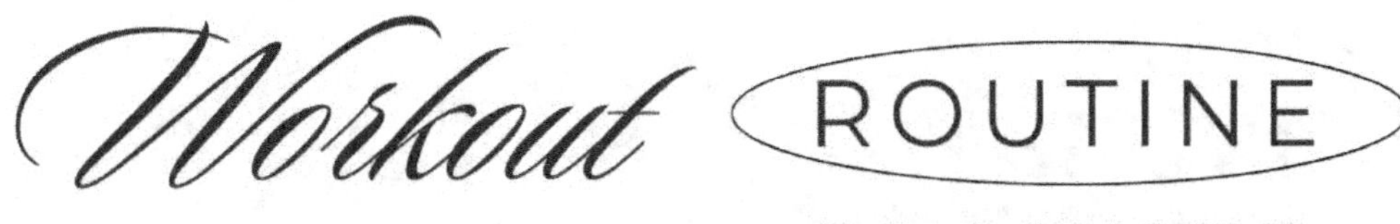

WEEK _______________

	WORKOUT	SOMETHING TO EAT	MY GOALS
Monday			

	WORKOUT	SOMETHING TO EAT	MY GOALS
Tuesday			

	WORKOUT	SOMETHING TO EAT	MY GOALS
Wednesday			

	WORKOUT	SOMETHING TO EAT	MY GOALS
Thursday			

	WORKOUT	SOMETHING TO EAT	MY GOALS
Friday			

	WORKOUT	SOMETHING TO EAT	MY GOALS
Saturday			

	WORKOUT	SOMETHING TO EAT	MY GOALS
Sunday			

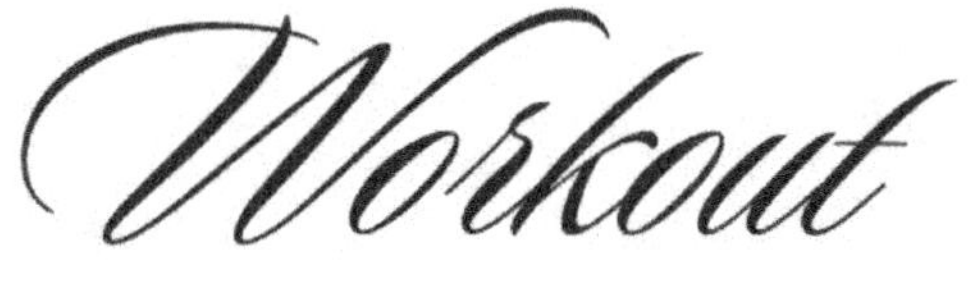

WEEK ________________

	WORKOUT	SOMETHING TO EAT	MY GOALS
Monday			

	WORKOUT	SOMETHING TO EAT	MY GOALS
Tuesday			

	WORKOUT	SOMETHING TO EAT	MY GOALS
Wednesday			

	WORKOUT	SOMETHING TO EAT	MY GOALS
Thursday			

	WORKOUT	SOMETHING TO EAT	MY GOALS
Friday			

	WORKOUT	SOMETHING TO EAT	MY GOALS
Saturday			

	WORKOUT	SOMETHING TO EAT	MY GOALS
Sunday			

Workout ROUTINE PLANNER

WEEK __________

Monday	WORKOUT	SOMETHING TO EAT	MY GOALS

Tuesday	WORKOUT	SOMETHING TO EAT	MY GOALS

Wednesday	WORKOUT	SOMETHING TO EAT	MY GOALS

Thursday	WORKOUT	SOMETHING TO EAT	MY GOALS

Friday	WORKOUT	SOMETHING TO EAT	MY GOALS

Saturday	WORKOUT	SOMETHING TO EAT	MY GOALS

Sunday	WORKOUT	SOMETHING TO EAT	MY GOALS

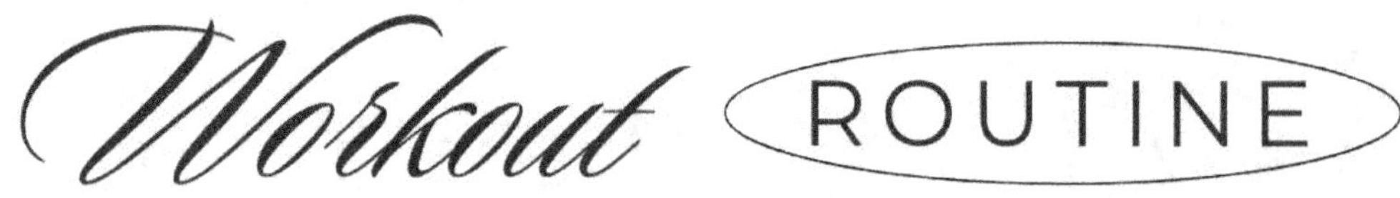

WEEK ______________

	WORKOUT	SOMETHING TO EAT	MY GOALS
Monday			

	WORKOUT	SOMETHING TO EAT	MY GOALS
Tuesday			

	WORKOUT	SOMETHING TO EAT	MY GOALS
Wednesday			

	WORKOUT	SOMETHING TO EAT	MY GOALS
Thursday			

	WORKOUT	SOMETHING TO EAT	MY GOALS
Friday			

	WORKOUT	SOMETHING TO EAT	MY GOALS
Saturday			

	WORKOUT	SOMETHING TO EAT	MY GOALS
Sunday			

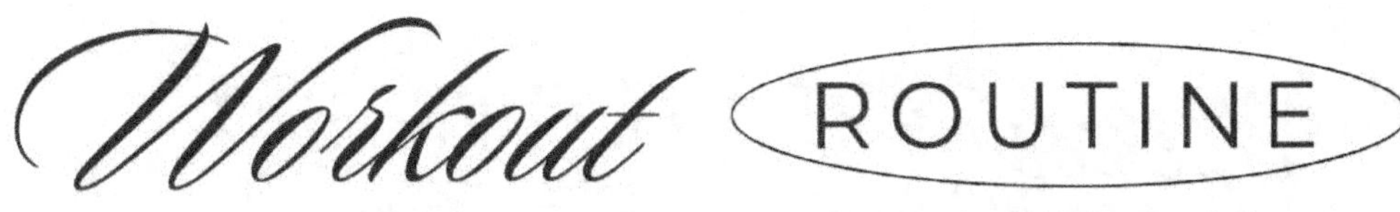

WEEK _______________

	WORKOUT	SOMETHING TO EAT	MY GOALS
Monday			

	WORKOUT	SOMETHING TO EAT	MY GOALS
Tuesday			

	WORKOUT	SOMETHING TO EAT	MY GOALS
Wednesday			

	WORKOUT	SOMETHING TO EAT	MY GOALS
Thursday			

	WORKOUT	SOMETHING TO EAT	MY GOALS
Friday			

	WORKOUT	SOMETHING TO EAT	MY GOALS
Saturday			

	WORKOUT	SOMETHING TO EAT	MY GOALS
Sunday			

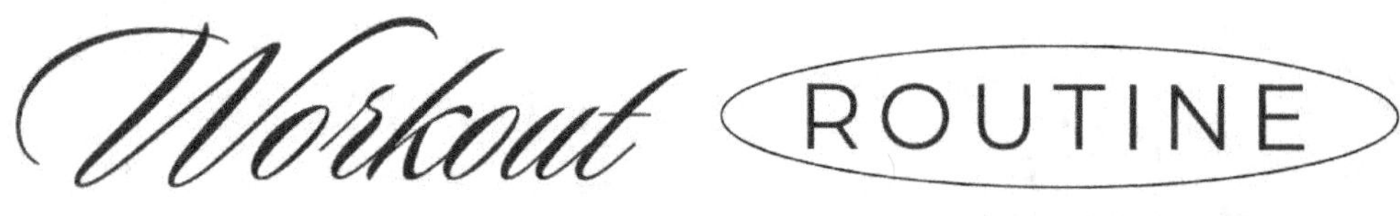

Workout ROUTINE PLANNER

WEEK ______________

	WORKOUT	SOMETHING TO EAT	MY GOALS
Monday			

	WORKOUT	SOMETHING TO EAT	MY GOALS
Tuesday			

	WORKOUT	SOMETHING TO EAT	MY GOALS
Wednesday			

	WORKOUT	SOMETHING TO EAT	MY GOALS
Thursday			

	WORKOUT	SOMETHING TO EAT	MY GOALS
Friday			

	WORKOUT	SOMETHING TO EAT	MY GOALS
Saturday			

	WORKOUT	SOMETHING TO EAT	MY GOALS
Sunday			

Workout 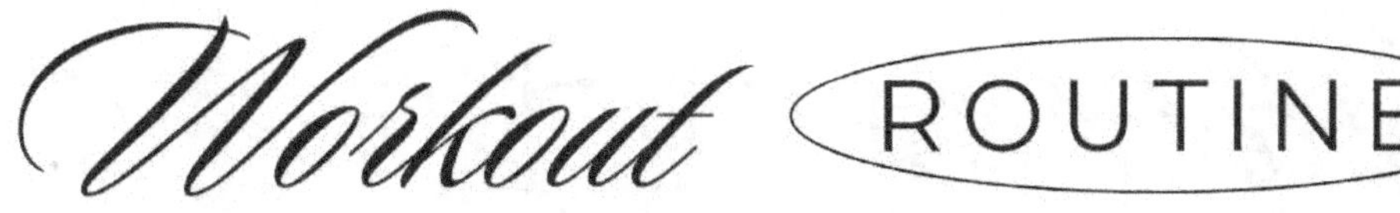 ROUTINE PLANNER

WEEK _______________

	WORKOUT	SOMETHING TO EAT	MY GOALS
Monday			

	WORKOUT	SOMETHING TO EAT	MY GOALS
Tuesday			

	WORKOUT	SOMETHING TO EAT	MY GOALS
Wednesday			

	WORKOUT	SOMETHING TO EAT	MY GOALS
Thursday			

	WORKOUT	SOMETHING TO EAT	MY GOALS
Friday			

	WORKOUT	SOMETHING TO EAT	MY GOALS
Saturday			

	WORKOUT	SOMETHING TO EAT	MY GOALS
Sunday			

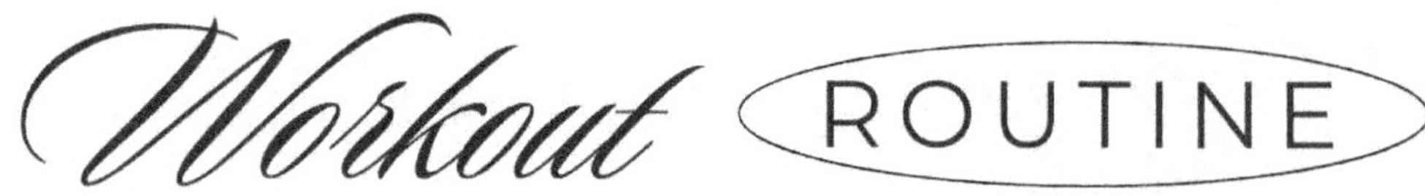

Workout (ROUTINE) PLANNER

WEEK _______________

Monday	WORKOUT	SOMETHING TO EAT	MY GOALS

Tuesday	WORKOUT	SOMETHING TO EAT	MY GOALS

Wednesday	WORKOUT	SOMETHING TO EAT	MY GOALS

Thursday	WORKOUT	SOMETHING TO EAT	MY GOALS

Friday	WORKOUT	SOMETHING TO EAT	MY GOALS

Saturday	WORKOUT	SOMETHING TO EAT	MY GOALS

Sunday	WORKOUT	SOMETHING TO EAT	MY GOALS

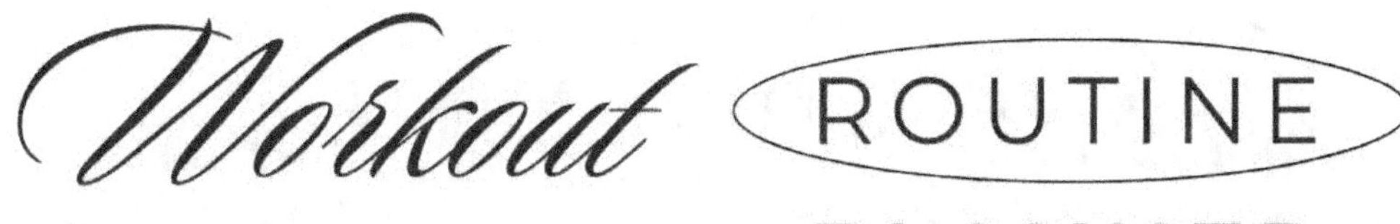

WEEK _______________

Monday	WORKOUT	SOMETHING TO EAT	MY GOALS

Tuesday	WORKOUT	SOMETHING TO EAT	MY GOALS

Wednesday	WORKOUT	SOMETHING TO EAT	MY GOALS

Thursday	WORKOUT	SOMETHING TO EAT	MY GOALS

Friday	WORKOUT	SOMETHING TO EAT	MY GOALS

Saturday	WORKOUT	SOMETHING TO EAT	MY GOALS

Sunday	WORKOUT	SOMETHING TO EAT	MY GOALS

Workout ROUTINE PLANNER

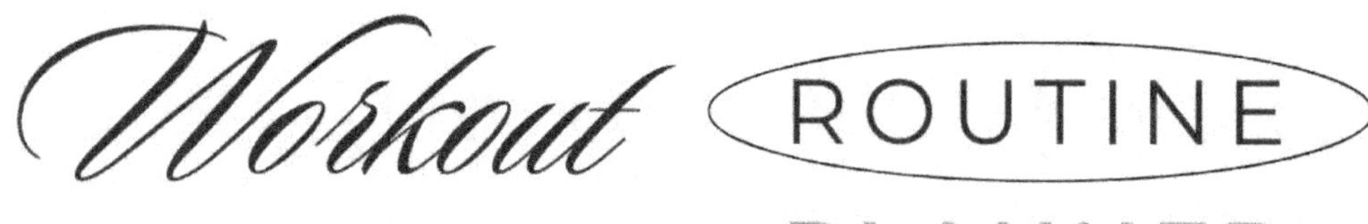

WEEK ________________

Monday	WORKOUT	SOMETHING TO EAT	MY GOALS

Tuesday	WORKOUT	SOMETHING TO EAT	MY GOALS

Wednesday	WORKOUT	SOMETHING TO EAT	MY GOALS

Thursday	WORKOUT	SOMETHING TO EAT	MY GOALS

Friday	WORKOUT	SOMETHING TO EAT	MY GOALS

Saturday	WORKOUT	SOMETHING TO EAT	MY GOALS

Sunday	WORKOUT	SOMETHING TO EAT	MY GOALS

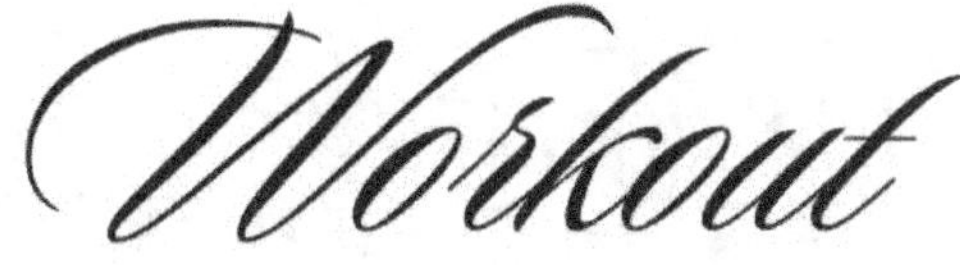

Workout ROUTINE PLANNER

WEEK ________________

Monday	WORKOUT	SOMETHING TO EAT	MY GOALS

Tuesday	WORKOUT	SOMETHING TO EAT	MY GOALS

Wednesday	WORKOUT	SOMETHING TO EAT	MY GOALS

Thursday	WORKOUT	SOMETHING TO EAT	MY GOALS

Friday	WORKOUT	SOMETHING TO EAT	MY GOALS

Saturday	WORKOUT	SOMETHING TO EAT	MY GOALS

Sunday	WORKOUT	SOMETHING TO EAT	MY GOALS

Workout 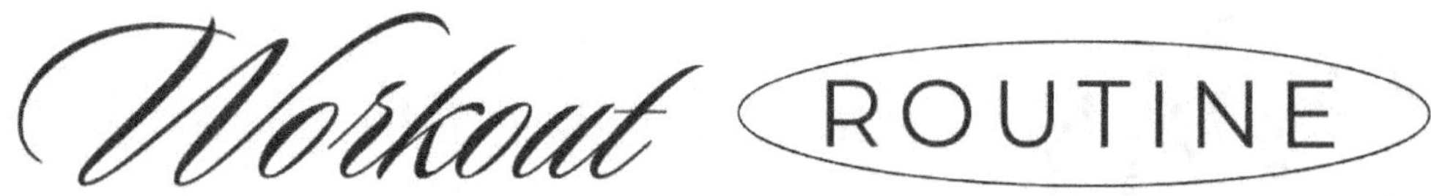 ROUTINE PLANNER

WEEK ______

	WORKOUT	SOMETHING TO EAT	MY GOALS
Monday			

	WORKOUT	SOMETHING TO EAT	MY GOALS
Tuesday			

	WORKOUT	SOMETHING TO EAT	MY GOALS
Wednesday			

	WORKOUT	SOMETHING TO EAT	MY GOALS
Thursday			

	WORKOUT	SOMETHING TO EAT	MY GOALS
Friday			

	WORKOUT	SOMETHING TO EAT	MY GOALS
Saturday			

	WORKOUT	SOMETHING TO EAT	MY GOALS
Sunday			